SCALP Acupuncture

CLINICAL TREATMENT

头针临床疗法

Sumiko Knudsen

Ph.D
Practitioner. DK

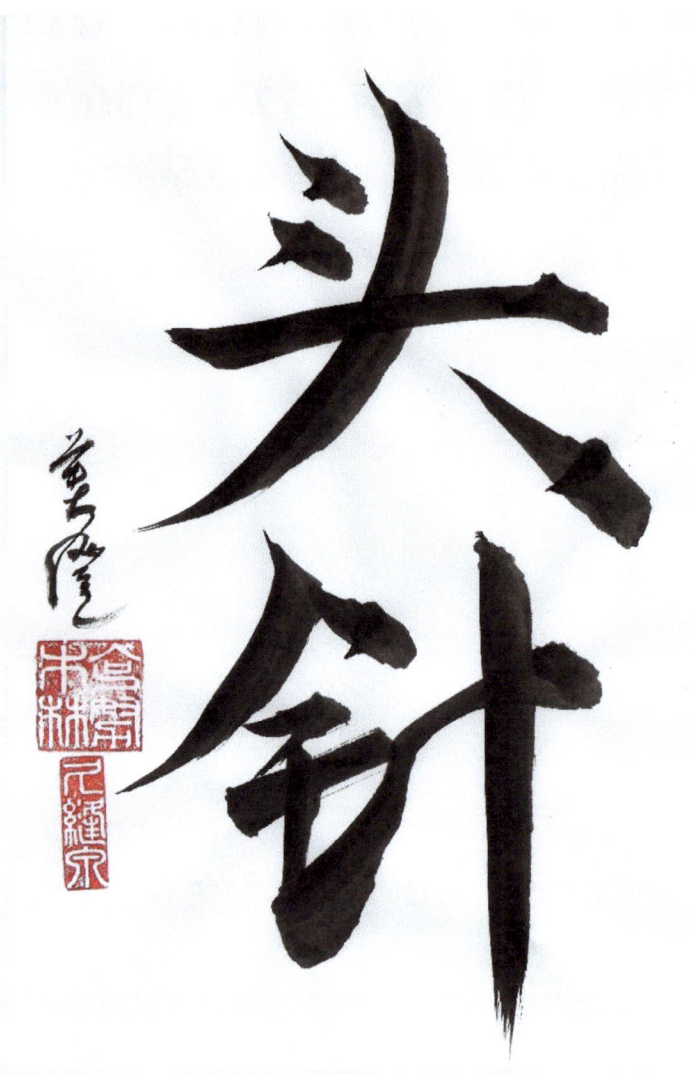

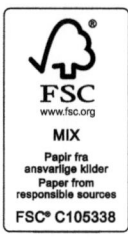
© 2021 Knudsen, Sumiko
Forlag: BoD – Books on Demand, Hellerup, Danmark
Tryk: BoD – Books on Demand, Norderstedt, Tyskland

ISBN: 9788743033707

CONTENTS

INTRODUCTION

Scalp Acupuncture is a therapy in which puncture of specific areas on the scalp is used to prevent or treat diseases.

The head is closely related to the meridians and Zang-Fu organs.
The six Yang meridians of hand and foot go through the head and face. The head is the gathering area of all the Yang.

All the meridians converge into the spinal cord and end at the brain. The meridian system can be used to treat hundreds of diseases and adjust the deficiency of the body.

Scalp Acupuncture was invented and developed through clinical practice by combining TCM and modern medicine. The stimulating areas of the scalp are defined by the location of the functional of the cerebral cortex.

Scalp Acupuncture often produces remarkable results by inserting a few needles.

Scalp Acupuncture works by stimulating the brain cells that are related to the impaired functions. The mechanism of Scalp Acupuncture is to "wake-up" the brain cells and to encourage the proper functioning of brain cells, to perform the lost function and to promote the brain system.

Scalp Acupuncture areas are often used in the rehabilitation of paralysis due to stroke, multiple sclerosis, and Parkinson's disease, etc.

Scalp Acupuncture is safe and effective.

Sumiko Knudsen 克努森澄子

Brodmann areas

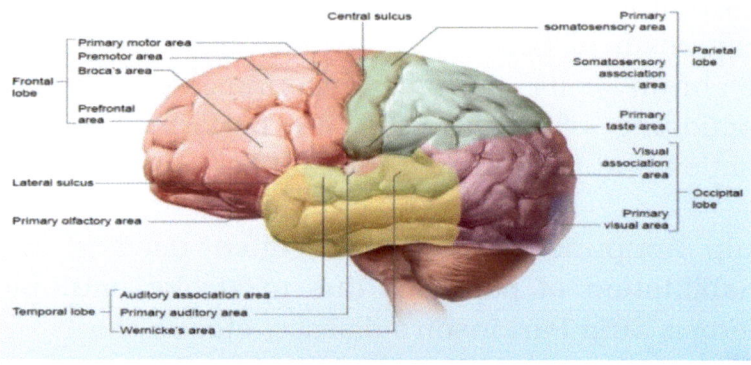

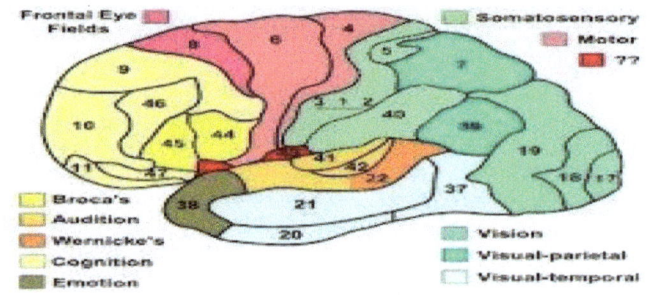

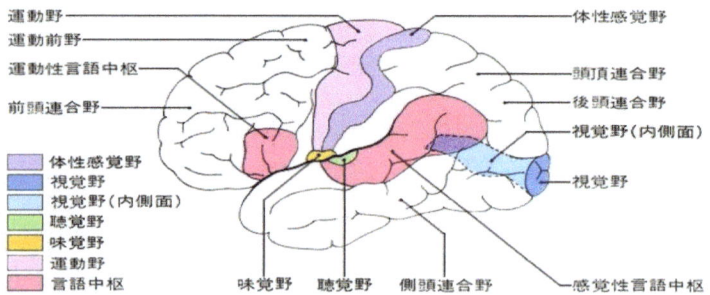

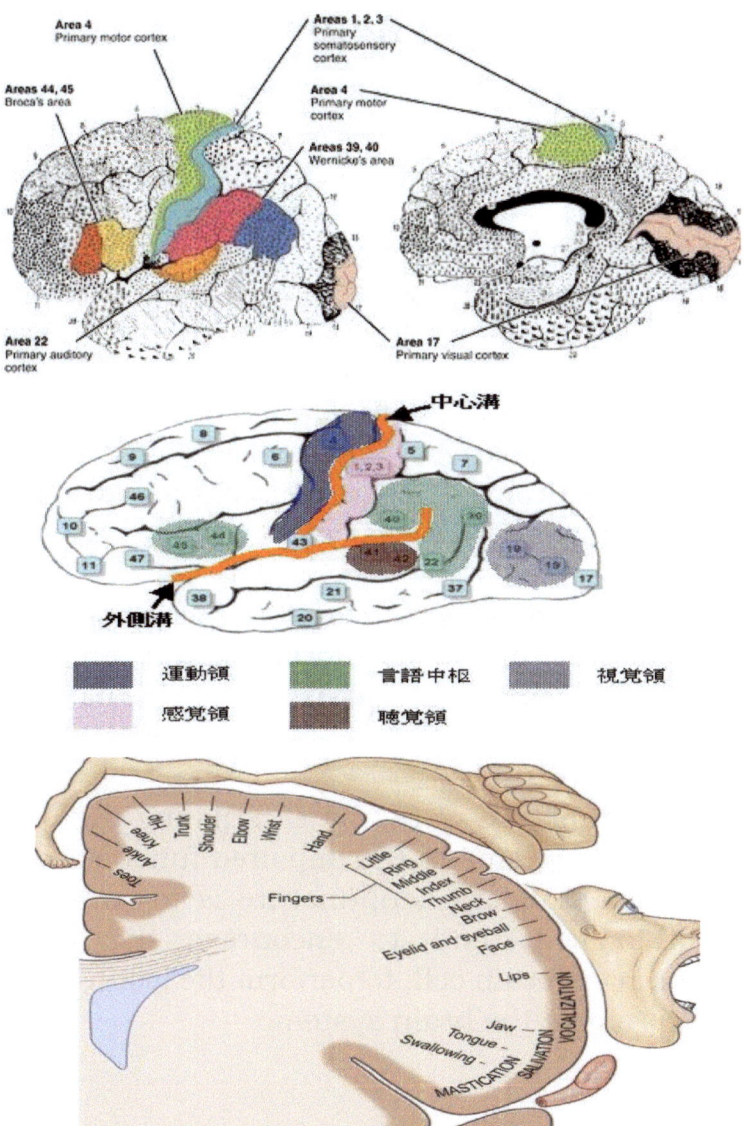

Chapter 1. Scalp Acupuncture Therapy

Scalp Acupuncture is Neuro Acupuncture, and the treatment is based on Traditional Chinese Acupuncture and neurology.

Clinical indications for treatment by Scalp Acupuncture are Aphasia, Paralysis, Parkinson's Disease, Multiple Sclerosis, Traumatic Brain Injury, Motor Neuron Diseases, Phantom Limb Syndrome, Meniere's Syndrome, Post-traumatic Stress disorder, Chorea, Alzheimer's Disease etc.

Through the central nervous and endocrine systems, the structural, metabolic, hormonal and energetic functions of the brain are accessible at specific areas of the scalp surface.

Scalp Acupuncture works by stimulating the brain cells that are related to the impaired functions. The mechanism of Scalp Acupuncture is to "wake-up" the brain cells and to encourage the proper functioning of brain cell, to perform the lost function and to promote the brain system.

The head is closely related to the meridians and Zang-Fu organs.

The six Yang meridians of hand and foot go through the head and face. The head is the gathering area of all the Yang.

All the meridians converge into the spinal cord and end at the brain. The meridian system can be used to treat hundreds of diseases and adjust the deficiency of the body.

Scalp acupuncture was invented and developed through clinical practice by combining TCM and modern medicine. The stimulating areas of the scalp are defined by the location of the functional area of the cerebral cortex.

I. Division of Stimulation Areas and Function

1. Standard Lines 标定线

There are two standard lines that are used to divide the stimulating areas.

1) The antero-posterior midline 前后正中线:

The midline connecting the midpoint between the two eyebrows with the lower border of the tip of the external occipital tuberosity across the vertex.

2) Eyebrow-occiput line 眉枕线:

The line connecting the midpoint of the superior border of the eyebrow with the tip of the external occipital tuberosity horizontally along the lateral side of the head.

Fig.1 shows the following.

1) Anterio-posterior midline 前后正中线
2) Midpoint of the superior border of eyebrow 眉上缘中点
3) Midpoint between eyebrows 眉间
4) Eyebrow occiput line 眉枕线
5) External occipital tuberosity 枕外粗隆

1.1 Scalp Acupuncture Diagram

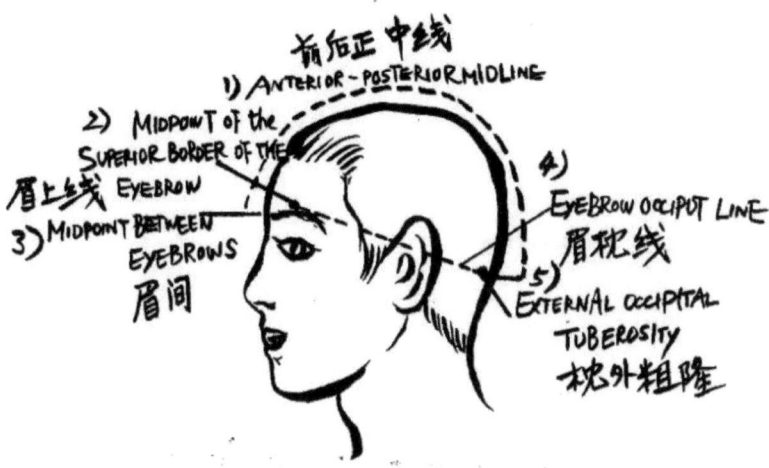

Fig. 1 Standard lines 标定线

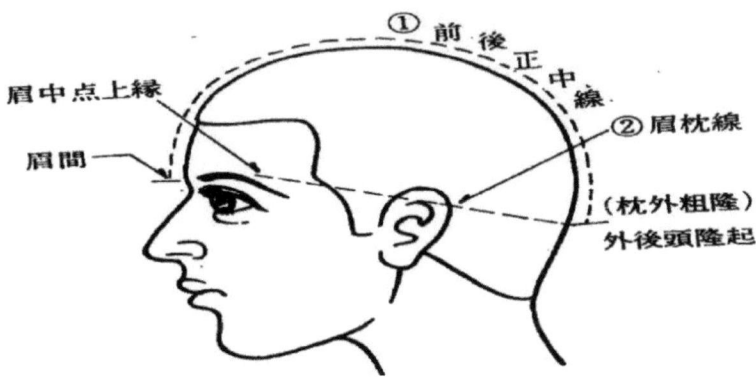

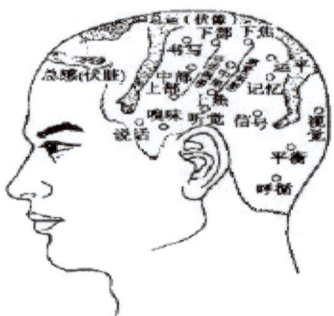

Fig. 2 Brodmann areas

2. Nerve System

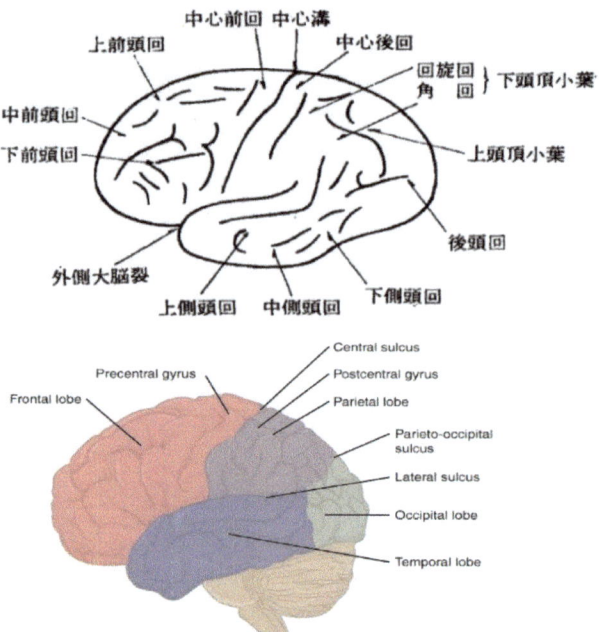

Fig. 3 Outer side

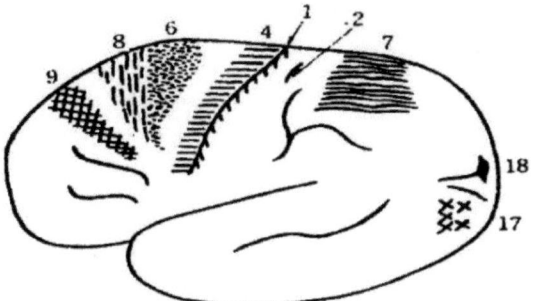

Fig. 4 Brodmann areas

Somatosensory cognition
体性感覚認知

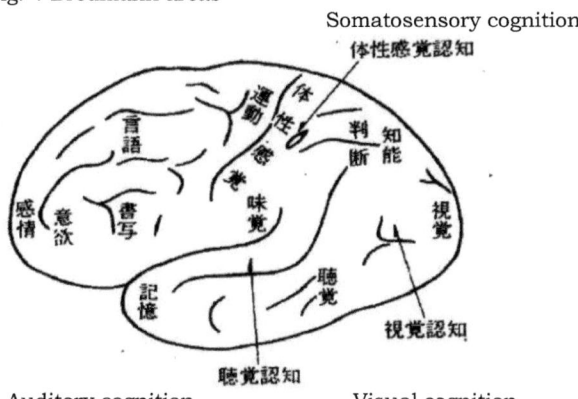

Auditory cognition   Visual cognition

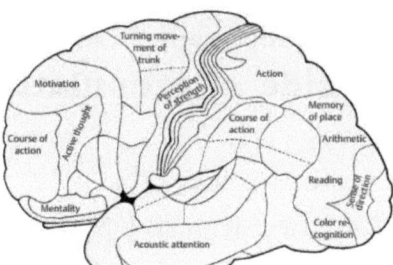

Fig. 5 Localization of Cerebral Cotex function

Brodmann areas is a morphological division of the cerebral cortex.

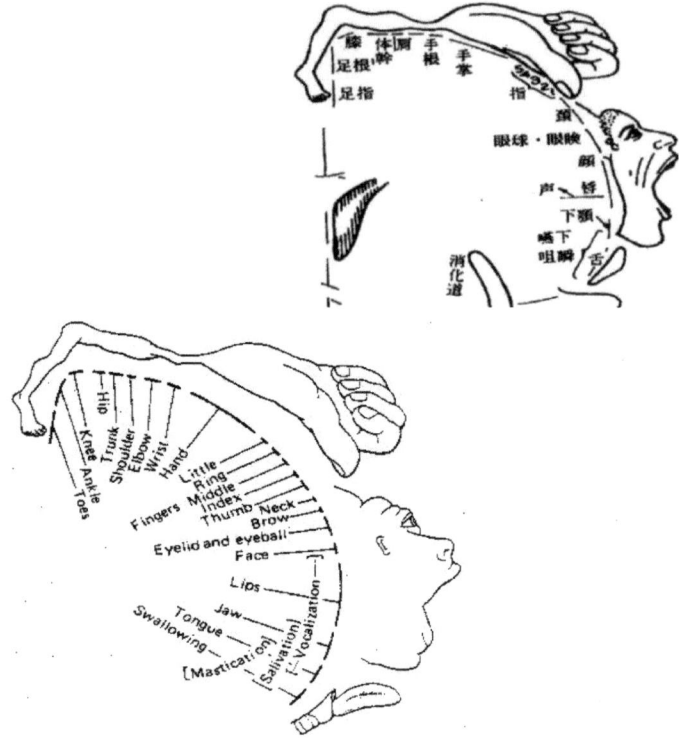

Fig. 6 Brodmann areas

3. Lateral side of stimulating area 侧面刺激区

- The motor area 运动区
- The sensory area 感觉区
- The chorea and tremor controlling area

- 舞蹈震颤控制区
- Vascular dilation and constriction area
- 血管扩张和收缩区
- The vertigo and auditory area 晕听区
- The second speech area 言语二区
- The third speech area 言语三区
- The usage area 运用区

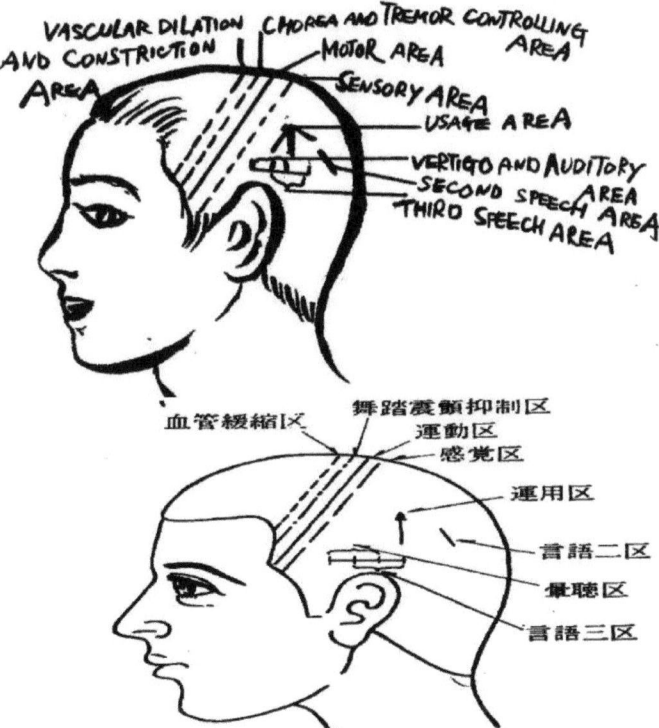

Fig. 2 Lateral side of stimulating area 侧面刺激区

(1) The motor area 运动区

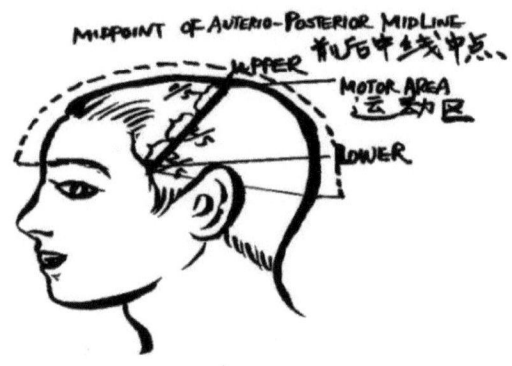

Fig. 2-1 Location of Motor area 运动区定位

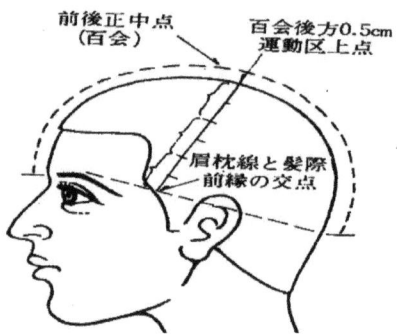

- Location

  0.5 cm posterior to the midpoint of anteroposterior midline as the upper point, and the intersect of the eyebrow-occiput line and the anterior border of the temple, the connecting line between these two points is the motor area.

- Indications
  Motor disturbance.

  1) Upper 1/5: To treat lower limb paralysis.
  2) Middle 2/5: To treat upper limb paralysis.
  3) Lower 2/5: To treat facial paralysis, motor aphasia, hyper salivation, disorder of pronunciation.

(2) The sensory area 感觉区

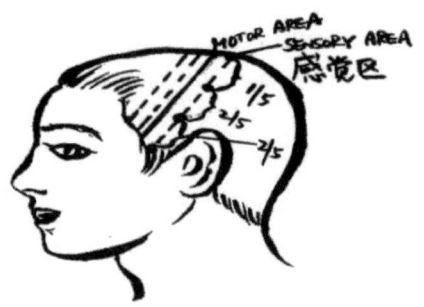

Fig. 2-2 Lateral side of Sensory area 感觉区

- Location
  The parallel line. 1.5cm behind the motor area.

- Indications
  Sensory disturbance.
  1) Upper 1/5: To treat lower limb pain, numbness, and abnormal sensation of the contralateral side in the back and leg, occipital headache, pain of the neck and nape, and tinnitus.

  2) Middle 2/5: To treat upper limb pain, numbness, and abnormal sensation of the contralateral arm.
  3) Lower 2/5: To treat numbness and pain of the contralateral side in the head and face.

(3) The chorea and tremor controlling area
舞蹈震颤控制区

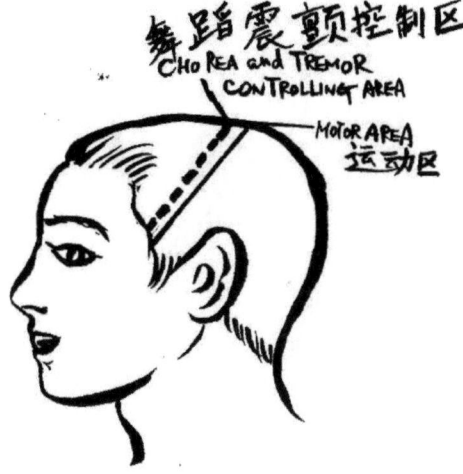

Fig. 2-3 Chorea and tremor controlling area 舞蹈震颤控制区

- Location
  Parallel line. 1.5 cm to the motor area.

- Indications
  To treat Chorea, Parkinson's disease.

(4) Vascular dilation and constriction area
血管扩张和收缩区

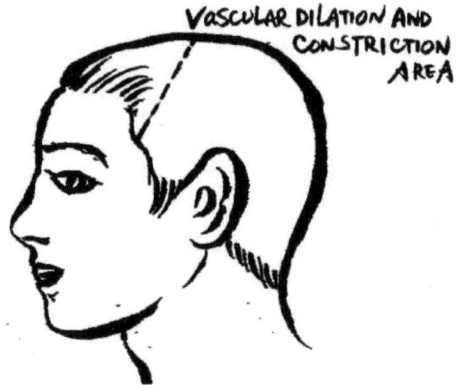

Fig. 2-4 Vascular dilation and constriction area 血管扩张和收缩
区

- Location
  Parallel line. 1.5 cm to the front of the chorea
  and tremor controlling area.

- Indications
  Hypertension and cortical edema.
  1) Upper 1/2: To treat upper limb cutaneous
  edema.
  2) Lower 1/2: To treat lower limb cutaneous
  edema.

Edema may be seen in patients with numbness and
paralyzed limbs. This type of edema is hepatobiliary
malnutrition because of hypersensitivity.

(5) The vertigo and auditory area 晕听区

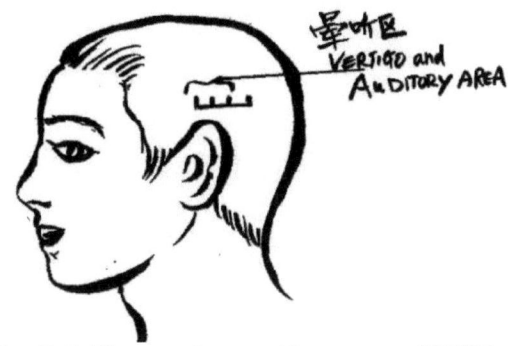

Fig. 2-5 The vertigo-auditory area 晕听区

- Location
  1.5 cm directly above the tip of auricular apex as the midpoint of 4cm horizontal in length.

- Indications
  To treat tinnitus, loss of hearing, auditory vertigo, dizziness, Meniere's syndrome.

(6) The second speech area 言语二区

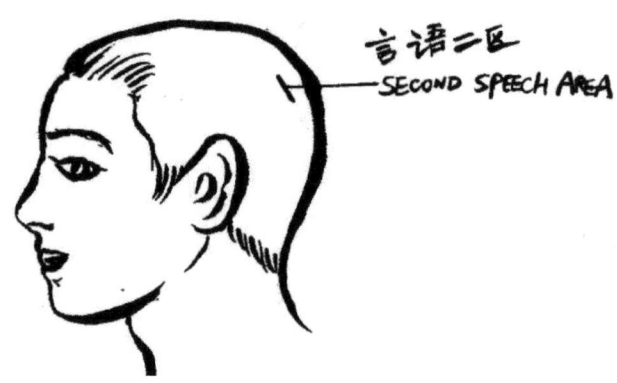

Fig. 2-6 The second speech area 言语二区

- Location
  This area is a 3 cm straight line, starting from a point 2 cm posterior and inferior to the parietal tubercle, parallel to the antero-posterior midline.

- Indications
  Aphasia.

(7) The third speech area 言语三区

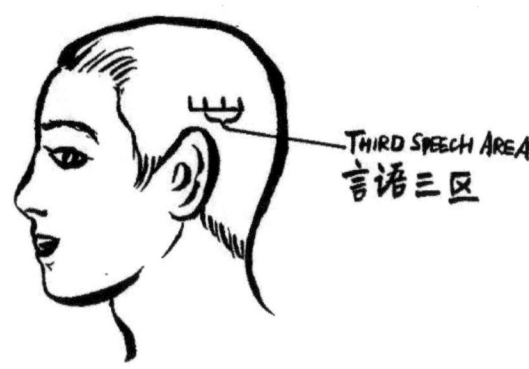

Fig. 2-7 The third speech area 言语三区

- Location
  Extending line backward from the midpoint of
  dizziness and auditory area, 4 cm in length.

- Indications
  Sensory aphasia.

(8) The usage/application area 运用区

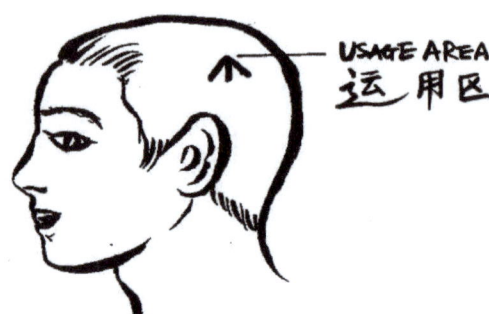

Figure 2-8 The usage area 运用区

- Location
  Take the parietal tubercles a starting point, draw a vertical line from the point, at the same time draw the other two lines from the point separately forwards and backwards, at 40 degree angle with the vertical line, each of the three lines is 3 cm long.

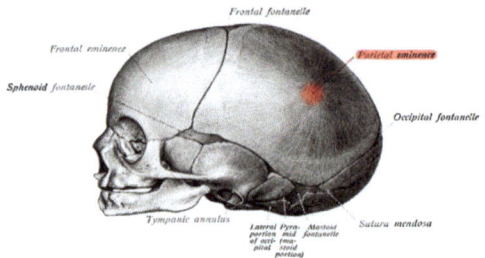

- Indications
  Apraxia (inability to perform particular actions).

4. Stimulation areas of the posterior side of the head 后面刺激区

- Foot Motor Sensory area 足运感区
- Second Speech area
- Optic area 视区
- Balance area 平衡区

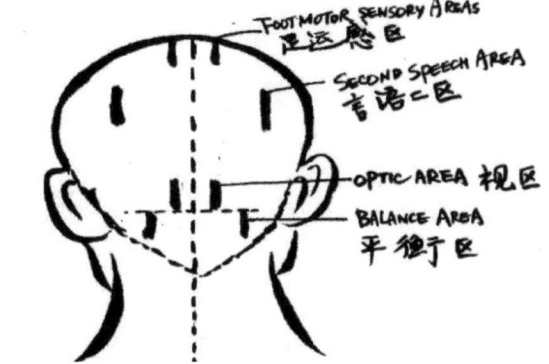

Fig. 3 Stimulation areas of the posterior side of the head 后面刺激区

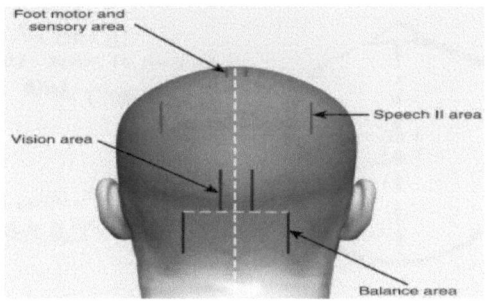

(1) The Foot motor sensory area 足运感区

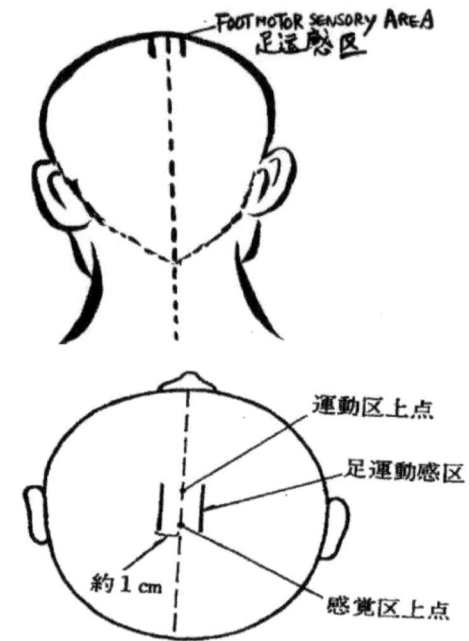

Fig. 4-1 The foot motor sensory area 足运感区

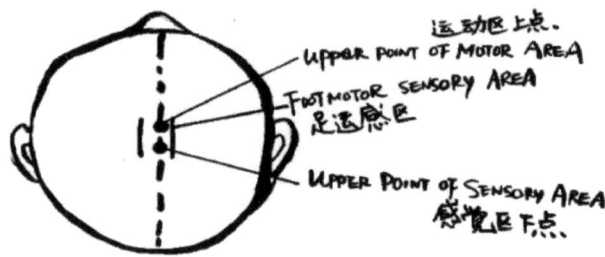

Fig.4-1A Viewed from the Top of the Head

- Location
Two parallel lines 1 cm beside the anterio-posterior midline, 3 cm in length, from a point 1 cm to the front of the upper end of motor area to a point 1 cm to the back of the upper end of sensory area.

- Indications
1) Main treatment: Lower limb pain, numbness, paralysis.

2) Secondary treatment: Acute lumbar sprain, cerebro-cortical polyuria, nocturia, prolapse of the uterus.

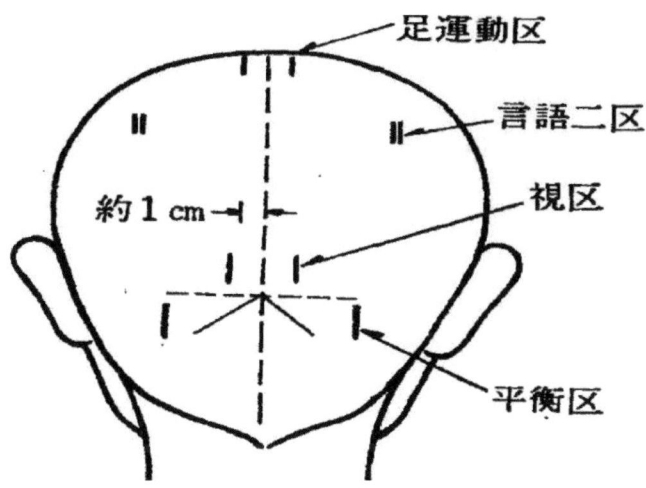

(2) The Optic area 视区

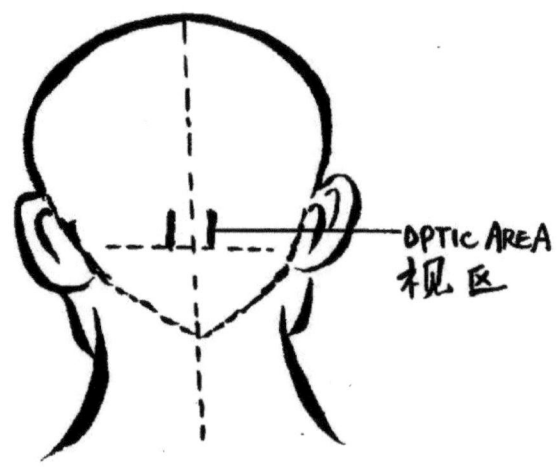

Fig. 4-2 The optic area 视区

- Location
  Two 4 cm parallel lines to the antero-posterior midline, 1 cm beside the external occipital protuberance.

- Indications
  Cerebro-cortical visual disturbance.

(3) The Balance area 平衡区

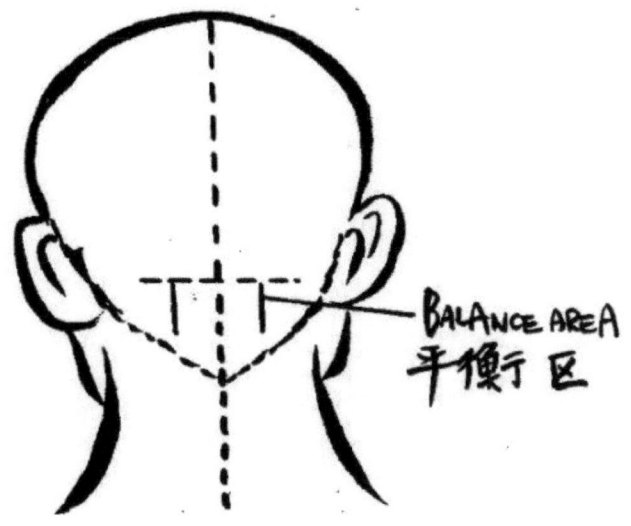

Fig. 4-3 The balance area 平衡区

- Location
  4 cm straight line downwards, parallel to the antero-posterior midline, 3.5 cm evenly beside the external occipital protuberance.

- Indications
  Equilibrium disturbance caused by cerebellum disease.

5. Stimulation areas of the anterior side of the head

- Thoracic Cavity area 胸腔区
- Stomach area 胃区
- Reproductive area 生殖区
- Intestine area 肠区
- Liver and Gallbladder area 肝胆区

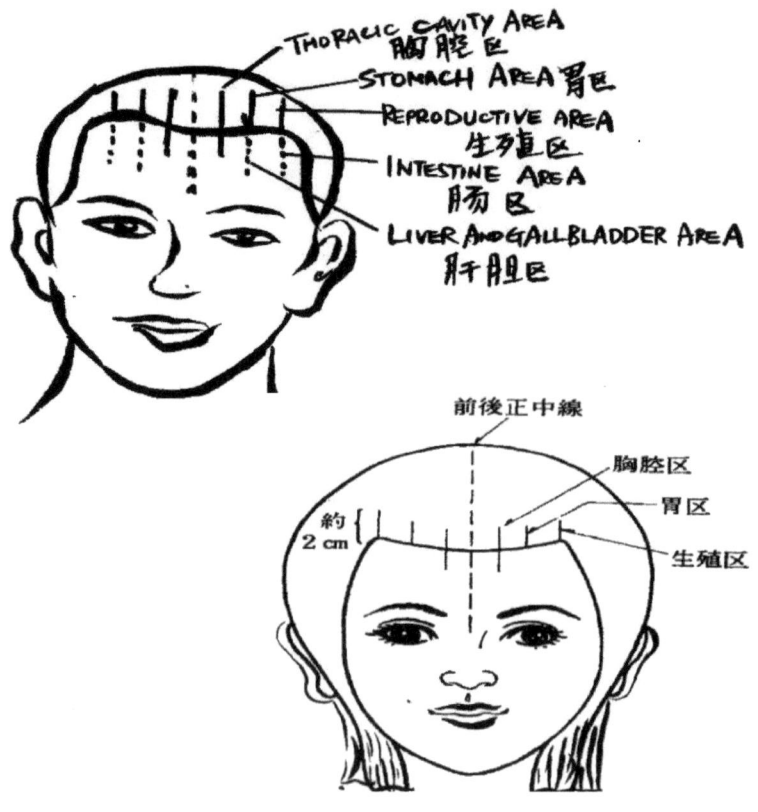

(1) Stomach area 胃区

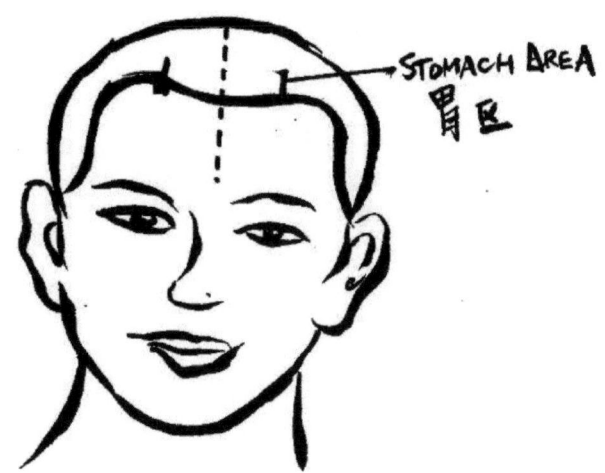

Fig. 5-1 Stomach area 胃区

- Location
  Two parallel vertical lines of 2 cm in length directly above the centre of pupils from the anterior hair border.

- Indications
  Gastric and epigastric pain.

(2) Liver and gallbladder area 肝胆区

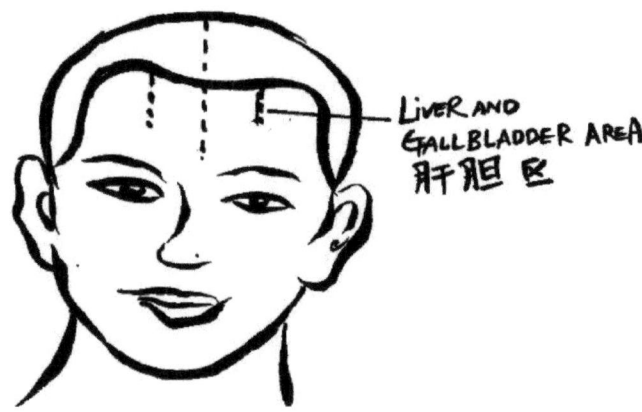

Fig. 5-2 Liver and gallbladder area 肝胆区

- Location
  Extending the stomach area to downward for 2 cm.

- Indications
  Upper stomach pain due to liver and gallbladder disorder.

(3) Thoracic cavity area 胸腔区

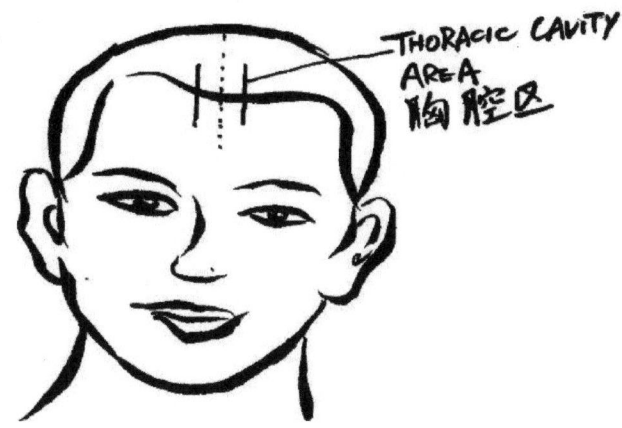

Fig. 5-3 Thoracic cavity area 胸腔区

- Location
  Two 4 cm parallel line between median line and the stomach area, with 2 cm above and 2 cm below the anterior hairline.

- Indications
  Chest pain, palpitation, angina pectoris, asthma, bronchitis, edema, hiccup.

(4) Reproductive area 生殖区

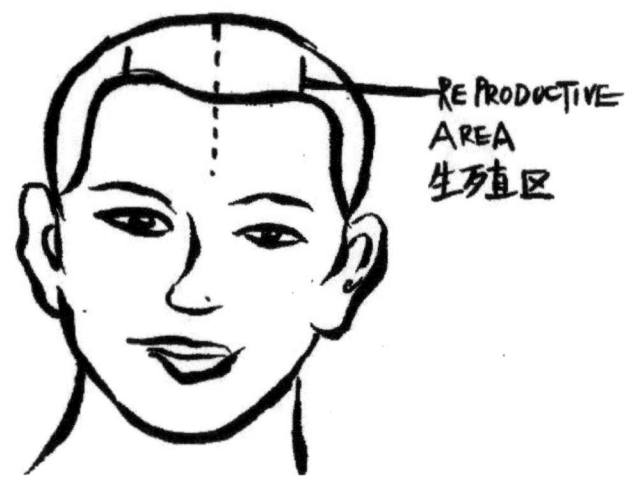

Fig. 5-4 Reproductive area 生殖区

- Location
  2 cm vertical lines, parallel to the frontal
  corner upward.

- Indications
  Dysfunctional uterine bleeding, leukorrhagia,
  polyuria due to diabetes mellitus.

(5) Intestine area 肠区

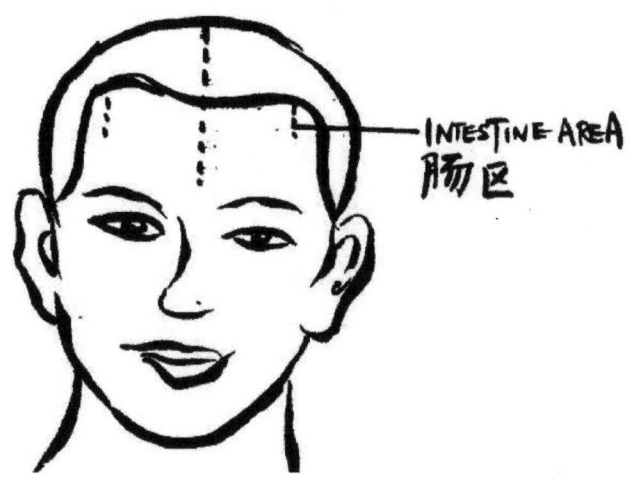

Fig. 5-5 Intestine area 肠区

- Location
  Extending the reproductive area on both sides
  downward for 2 cm.

- Indications
  Pain of lower abdomen.

II. Standard nomenclature of Chinese Scalp Acupuncture line 标准术语

1. Forehead Region

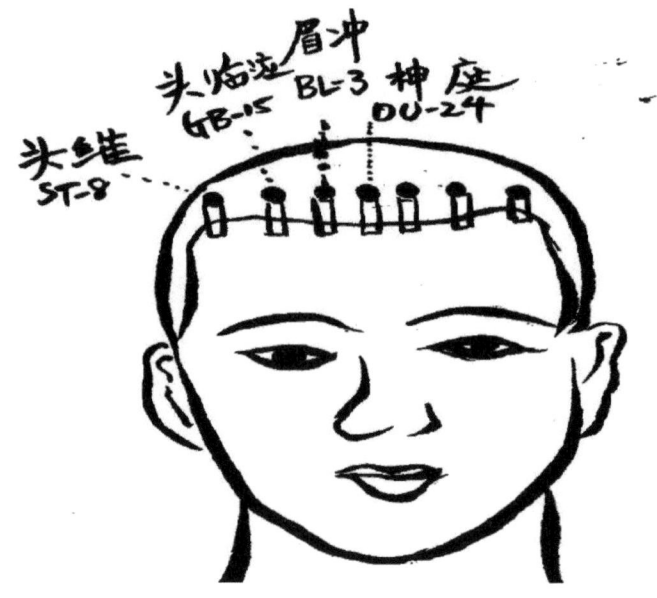

(1) Middle Line of Forehead (MS-1)

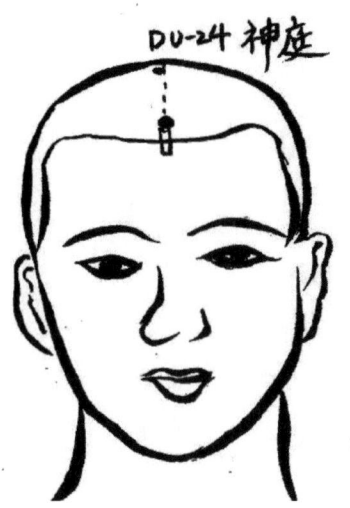

DU-24 神庭

- Location
  At the middle of the frontal area, 1 cun long from DU-24 (Shenting 神庭), (0.5 cun above the hair line) straight down along the DU meridian.

- Indications
  Mental disorders, epilepsy, diseases of head, nose, tongue, throat.

(2) Line 1 Lateral to Forehead (MS-2)

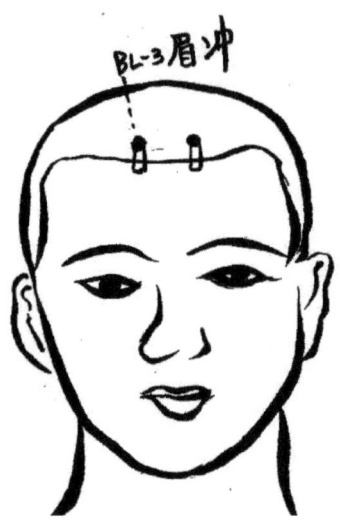

- Location
  1 cun long from BL-3 (Meichong 眉冲) (0.5 cun above the hair line) straight down along BL meridian.

- Indications
  Disorders is located upper jiao. Lung, bronchus, heart, angina, pectoris, allergic asthma, insomnia.

(3) Line 2 Lateral to Forehead (MS-3)

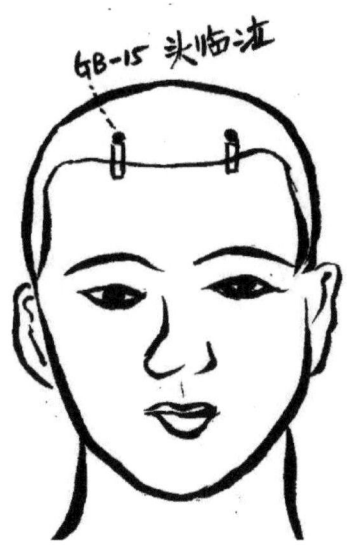

- Location
  1 cun long from GB-15 (Toulinqi 头临泣)
  straight down along the GB meridian.

- Indications
  Disorder is located middle jiao. Stomach, liver,
  gallbladder. Gastritis, gastric ulcer, duodenal
  ulcer.

(4) Line 3 Lateral to Forehead (MS-4)

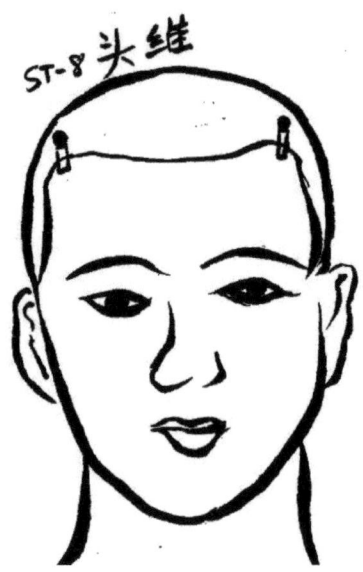

- Location
  1 cun long from the point 0.75 cun medial to
  ST-8 (touwei 头维) straight down.

- Indications
  Disorder is located lower jiao. Kidney, urinary
  bladder, genetic system. Dysfunctional uterine
  bleeding, impotence, seminal emission,
  prolapse of uterus, frequent urination, urgent
  urination.

2. Vertex Region

(5) Middle Line of Vertex (MS-5)

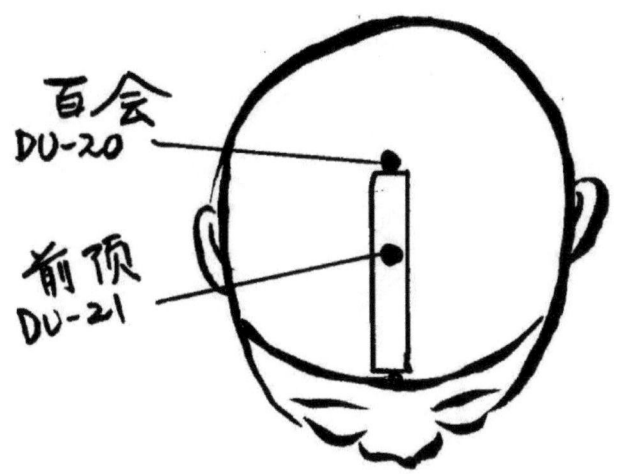

- Location
  From DU-20 (Baihui 百会) to DU-21 (Qianding 前顶) (1.5 cun) along the DU meridian, Governor Vessel.

- Indications
  Low back pain, leg pain, lower limb paralysis, numbness and pain, prolapse of rectum, cortical polyuria, nocturnal enuresis.

(6) Anterior Oblique Line of Vertex-Temporal (MS-6)

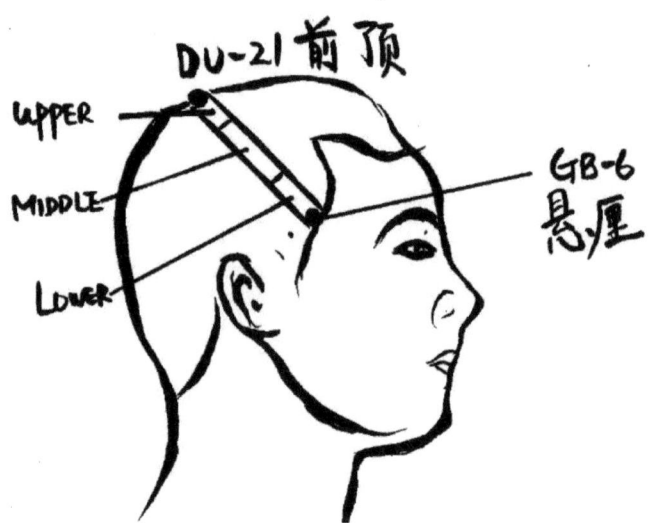

- Location
  From DU-21 (Qianding 前顶) obliquely to GB-6 (Xuanli 悬厘), passing across DU meridian, Governor vessel.

- Indications
  When the line is divided equally into five portions:

The upper 1/5:
lower limb paralysis, arthralgia.

The middle 2/5:
upper limb paralysis.

The lower 2/5:
disorder of head and face, facial paralysis, aphemia, salivation, aphasis, cerebral arteriosclerosis.

(7) Posterior Oblique Line of Vertex-Temporal (MS-7)

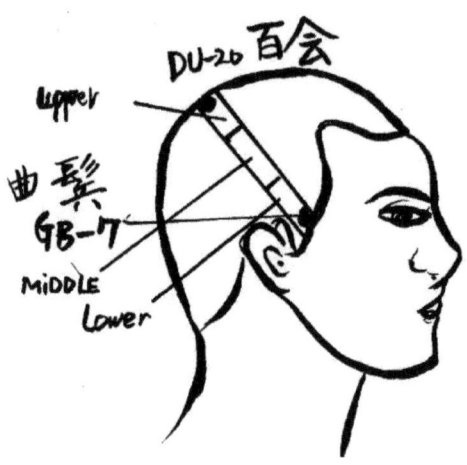

- Location
  From DU-20 (Baihui) obliquely to GB-7 (Qubin 曲鬓).

- Indications
  The upper 1/5:
  Sensory disturbance of lower limb.

  The middle 2/5:
  Sensory disturbance of upper limb.

  The lower 2/5:
  Sensory disturbance of head and face.

(8) Line 1 Lateral Vertex (MS-8)

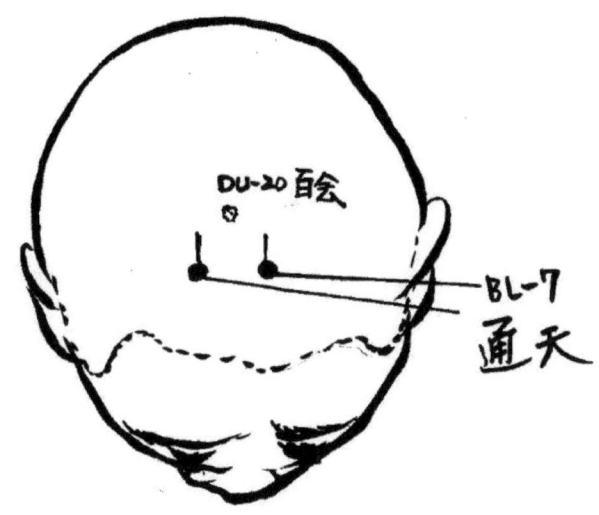

- Location
  1.5 cun lateral to middle line of vertex, 1.5 cun
  from BL-7 (Tongtian 通天), backward along the
  meridian.

- Indications
  Low back and leg pain, paralysis, numbness.

(9) Line 2 Lateral to Vertex (MS-9)

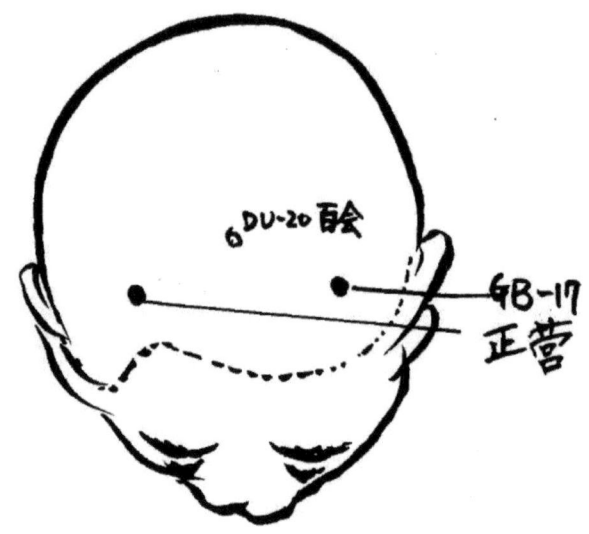

- Location
  2.25 cun lateral to middle line of vertex, 1.5 cun long from GB-17 (Zhengying 正营) backward along the meridian.

- Indications
  Disorders in shoulder, arm and hand paralysis, numbness, pain.

3. Temporal Region

(10) Anterior Temporal Line (MS-10)

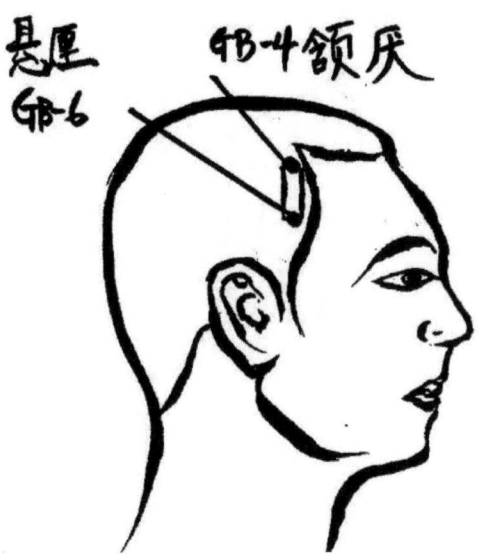

- Location
  From GB-4 (Hanyan 頷厌) to GB-6 (Xuanli 悬厘).

- Indications
  Migraine, aphemia, aphasia, Bell's palsy.

(11) Posterior Temporal Line (MS-11)

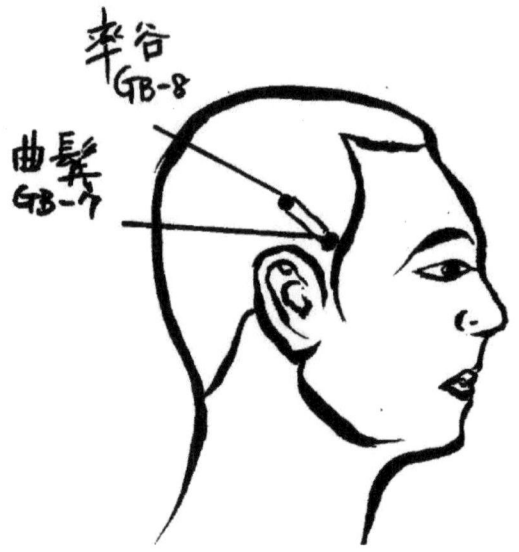

- Location
  From GB-8 (Shuaigu 率谷) to GB-7 (Qubin 曲
  鬢).

- Indications
  Migraine, vertigo, tinnitus, deafness.

4. Occipital Region

(12) Upper Middle Line of Occiput (MS-12)

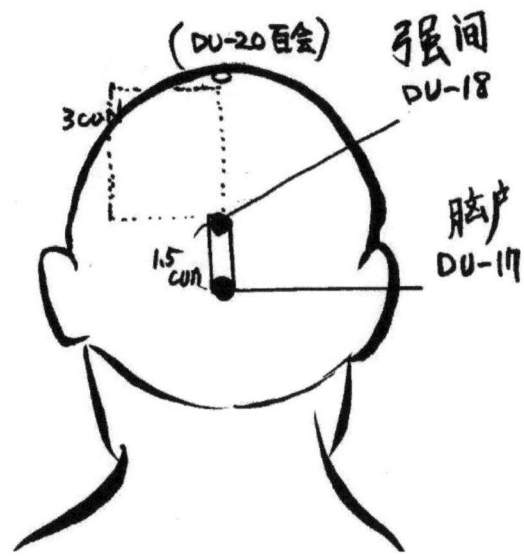

- Location
  From DU-18(Qiangjian 强间) to DU-17(Naohu
  脑户). 1.5cun long.

- Indications
  Various eye diseases.

(13) Upper Lateral Line of Occiput (MS-13)

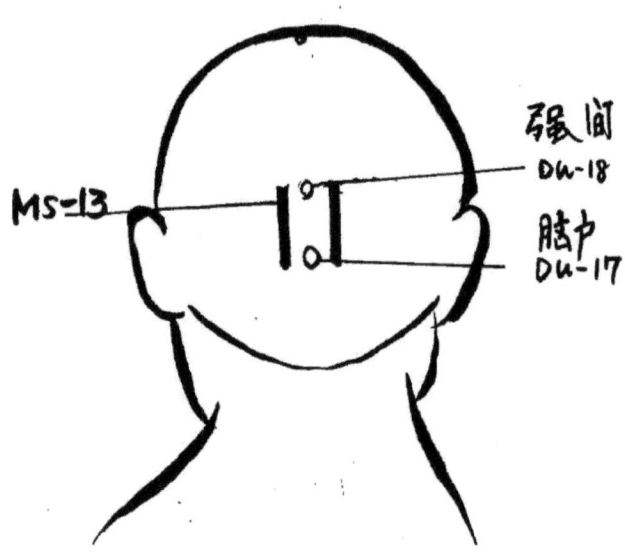

- Location
  0.5 cun lateral and parallel to upper middle line of occiput and belonging to the Bladder meridian.

- Indications
  Cortical visual disturbance, cataract myopia, lumbar muscle strain.

(14) Lower Lateral Line of Occiput (MS-14)

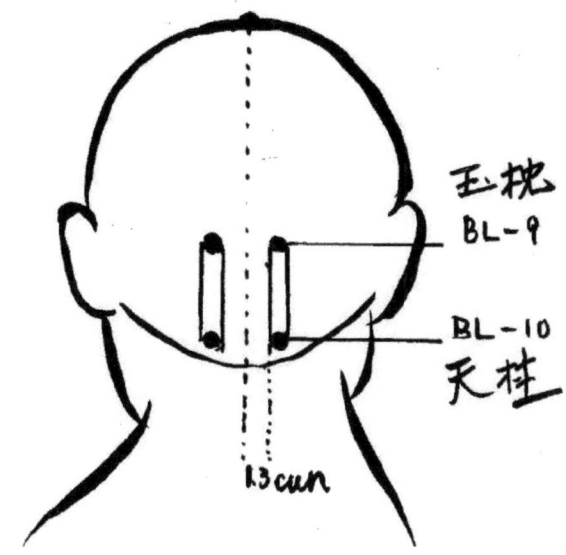

- Location
  From BL-9 (Yuzen 玉枕) to BL-10(Tianzhu 柱).

- Indications
  Cerebellum disorders, disequilibrium, occipital headache.

(15) Lower Curve zone of Occipital/ Bottom of the Skull Zone

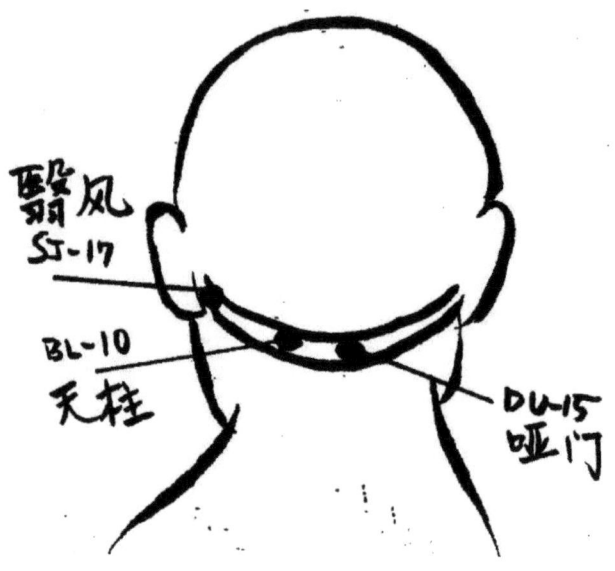

- Location
  From DU-15 (Yamen 哑门), BL-10 (Tianzhu 天柱) to SJ-17 (Yifeng 翳风).

- Indications
  Migraine, pain of neck and shoulder, mental problem, epilepsy, Alzheimer, tinnitus, deafness, vertigo, hypertension.

Occipital Region

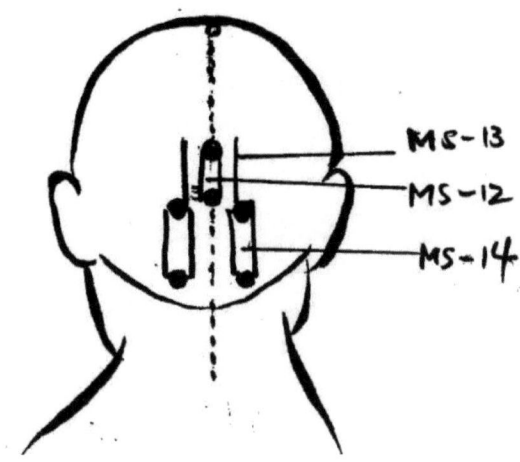

MS-13
MS-12
MS-14

Temporal Posterior Region

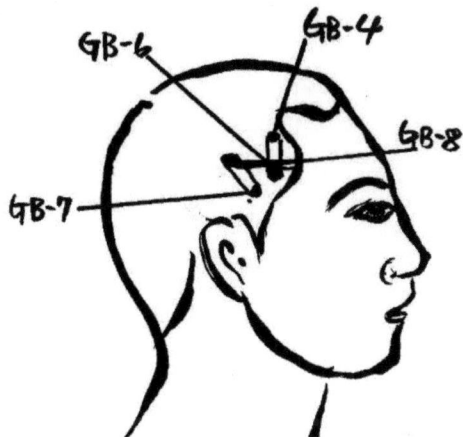

GB-6
GB-4
GB-8
GB-7

Temporal Posterior Oblique Region

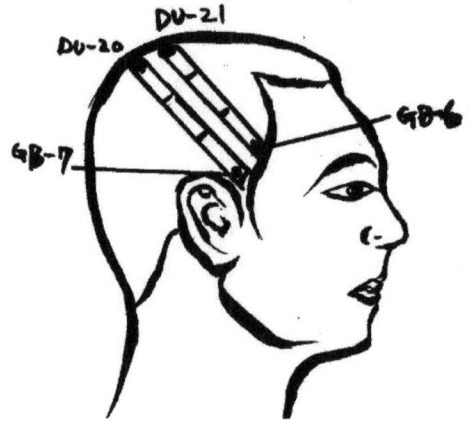

Chapter 2. Clinical Treatment
I. Cerebrovascular Disorders

1-1 Cerebral haemorrhage (Naochuxie 脑出血) on the right side.

- Symptom
  Arm movement impaired.
- Treatment
  1) Motor area on the left side.

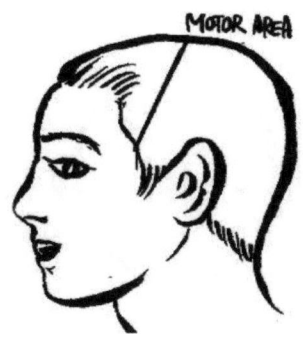

Lateral view

1-2 Cerebral Embolism (Naoshuansai 脑栓塞)

- Symptom
Cerebrovascular disease due to the blockade of the cerebral artery. Facial paralysis, monoplegia of the upper limbs, hemiplegia, aphasia, convulsion.

- Treatment
1) Motor area.
2) Sensory area.
3) Motor and sensory area of foot on the opposite side of the physical signs.

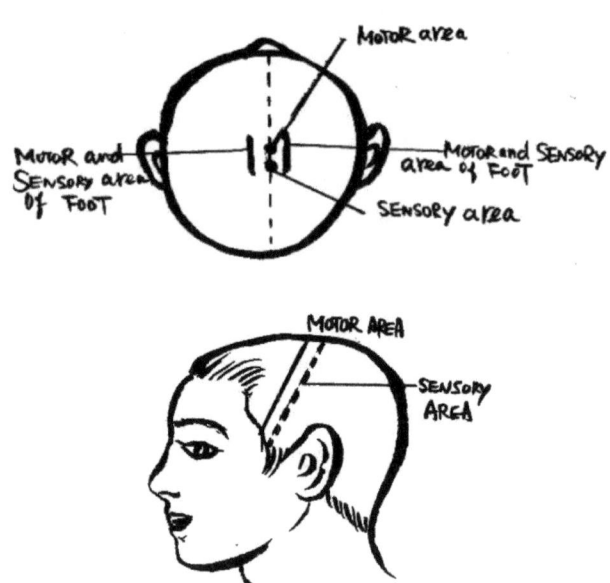

1-3 Cerebral Injury (Naosunshang 脑损伤)

- Symptom
  External trauma. Coma, hemiplegia, numbness and aphasia.

- Treatment
  1) Motor area.
  2) Motor and sensory area of foot on the opposite side of the physical symptoms.

1-4 Cerebral Thrombosis (Naoxueshuan 脑血栓)

- Symptom
  The pathological lesions in the cerebral blood vessels, such as atherosclerosis.
  Paralysis. Impairment of hands, dizziness, headache.

- Treatment
  1) Motor area.
  2) Sensory area.
  3) Motor and sensory area of foot on the contralateral side.

1-5 Intracranial Infection/Encephalitis (Luneiganran/naoyan 颅内感染/脑炎)

- Symptom
  Fever, convulsion, coma.

- Treatment
  1) Motor area.
  2) Optic areas on both sides.

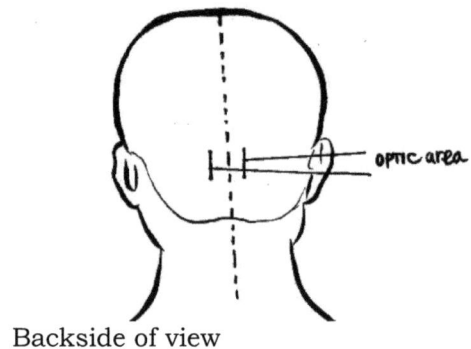

optic area

Backside of view

1-6 Hemiplegia on the right side after tuberculous meningitis (Jiehexingnaomoyanhouyouce 结核性脑膜炎后右侧偏瘫)

- Symptom

The movement of limbs and paralyses on the right side. Difficult to walk.

- Treatment
  1) Motor area.
  2) the motor and sensory area of foot on the left side of the body.

1-7 Toxic Encephalitis (Zhongduxingnaoyan 中毒性脑炎)

- Symptom
  Paralysis of limbs.

- Treatment
  1) Motor area.
  2) Motor and sensory area of foot on both sides.

1-8 Chorea (Wudaobing 舞蹈病)

- Symptom
  Involuntary movement of limbs.

- Treatment

Chorea and tremor controlling area on the opposite side of the symptoms, or on both sides.

1-9 Right Hemichorea (Youcepiancewudaozheng 右侧偏侧舞蹈症)

- Symptom
  Hemichorea is limited to limbs on one side of the body. It may be damage to the basal ganglia, and it can be chorea rheumatism. Weakness and involuntary movement of the limbs.

- Treatment
  Chorea and tremor controlling area on the left side.

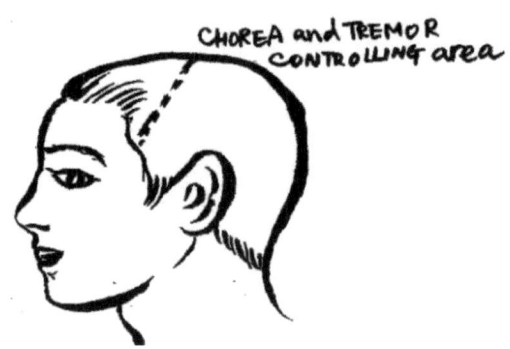

1-10 Right Hemichorea with slight Hemiplegia of right limbs (Youcepiantanbanyouzhiqingdupiantan 右侧偏袒伴右肢轻度偏袒)

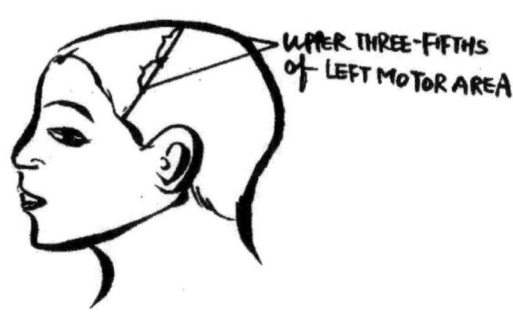

- Treatment
  1) Left chorea and tremor controlling area.
  2) Upper three-fifths of left motor area.
  3) Left motor and sensory area of foot.

1-11 Parkinson's disease (Pajinsenbing 帕金森病)

- Symptom
  Degenerative disease of the central nervous system. Tremor, muscular spasm and reduced action.

- Treatment
Chorea and tremor controlling area on both sides.

II. Peripheral nerves diseases

2-1 Facial Paralysis (Bell´s Palsy) (Miantan 面瘫)

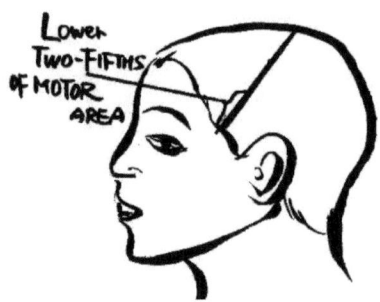

- Symptom
Inflammation of the facial nerve in stylomastoid foramen. Peripheral facial paralysis occurs on one side of the face.

- Treatment
Lower two-fifths of motor area on both sides.

2-2 Trigeminal Neuralgia (Sanchashenjingyan 三叉神经炎)

Trigeminal nerves are divided into three branches, which are supraorbital branch, maxillary branch and mandibular branch.

- Symptom
  It is manifested by sudden onset of facial pain, occurs in transient paroxysms, and just like cutting, burning and needling, which lasts for a few seconds or few minutes, and several times a day. It is accompanied by local spasm, lacrimation and salivation.

- Treatment
  1) Middle two-fifths: DU-20 (Baihui 百会) – GB7 (Qubin 曲鬓) zone.
  2) ST-8 (Touwei 头维)
  3) Upper of eyebrow and ST-7 (Xiaguan 下关)

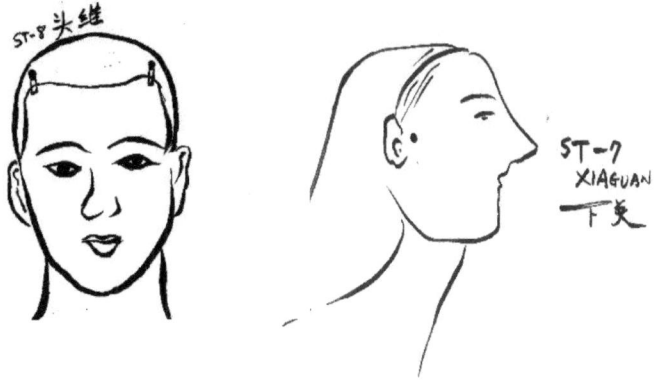

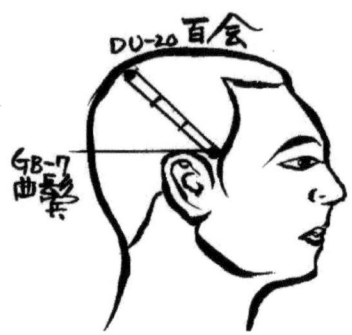

2-3 Herpes Zoster (Daizhuangpaozhen 带状 疱疹)

- Symptom
  Burning and pricking pain over the cutaneous area over the limbs and trunk. Covering somatomes innervated by the infected nerve roots with hypersensitivity to pain to the area.

- Treatment
  1) Sensory area.
  2) Motor and sensory area of foot on both sides.

2-4 Acute Infective Polyneuritis (Jixingganranxingduofaxingshenjingyan 急性感染性多发性神经炎)

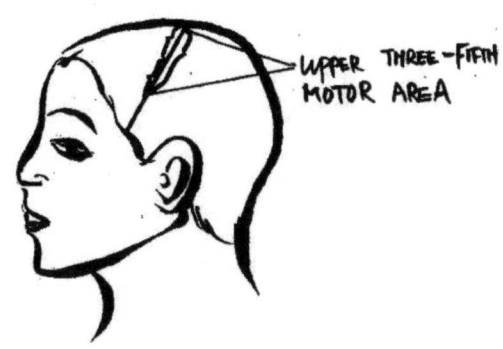

- Symptom
  Infection of the upper respiratory tract or the intestine. Body temperature is 38.5 degree.

- Treatment
  1) Upper three-fifths of motor area.
  2) Motor and sensory area of foot on both sides.

2-5 Sciatica (Zuogushengjingtong 坐骨神经痛)

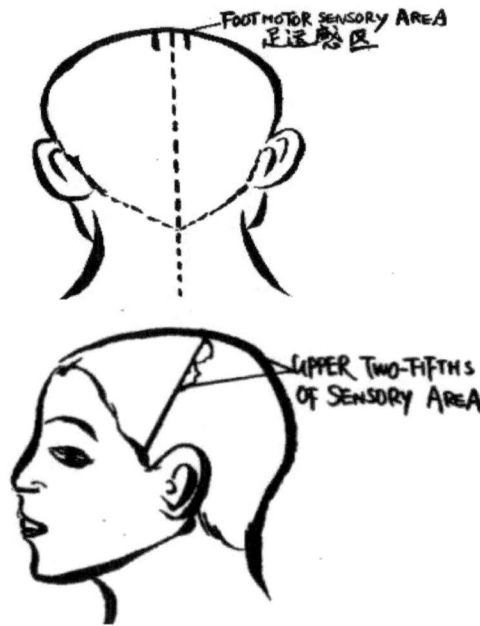

- Symptom
  The pain radiates from the lower back the posterior side of the thigh and side of the legs to the lateral border of the feet.

- Treatment
  1) Upper two-fifths of sensory area.
  2) Motor and sensory area of foot on both sides.

2-6 Schizpphrenja (Jingshenfenliezheng 精神分裂症)

- Symptom
  1. Heart and Liver Fire Exuberance
  Excitation, mania, not sleep whole night, glowering eyes, increasing the strength, yellow and brown urine, yellow tongue, and rapid pulse.

  2. Phlegm and Qi Stagnation
  Mental depression, dull eyes, anorexia, white greasy tongue, slippery pulse.

  3. Qi Stagnation and Blood Stasis
  Long-term mania, mental instability, delusion, insomnia, dull complexion, dry skin, purplish tongue, and deep pulse.

  4. Heat and Spleen Asthenia
  Depression, palpitation, palpitation, frighten, inactivity, light coloured tongue, and soft and weak pulse.

- Treatment
  1) DU-20 (Baihui 百会) -DU-21 (Qianding 前顶) zone.

2) BL-3 (Meichong 眉冲)

3) GB-15 (Toulinqi 头临泣)

4) DU-19 (Houding 后顶) -DU-18 (qiangjiang 强间) zone

5) DU-15 (Yamen 哑门) - SJ-17 (Yifeng 翳风) - BL-10 (Tianzhu 天柱) zone

6) Upper eyebrow

2-7 Mania (Zaokuang燥狂)

- Treatment

  1) DU-20 (Baihui 百会) -DU-21(Qianding 前顶) zone.

  2) BL-3 (Meichong 眉冲)

  3) GB-15 (Toulinqi 头临泣)

  4) DU-19 (Houding 后顶) -DU-18 (Qiangjiang 强间) zone

  5) DU-15 (Yamen 哑门) -SJ-17 (Yifeng 翳风) - BL-10 (Tianzhu 天柱) zone

6) Upper eyebrow

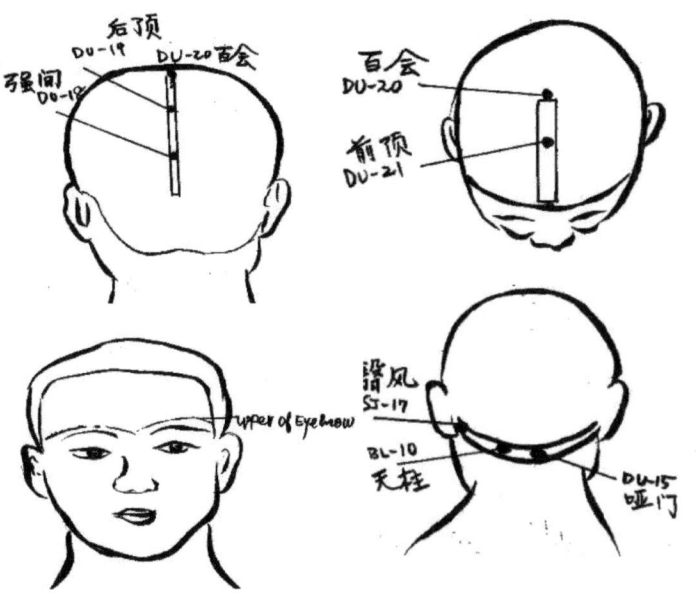

2-8 Dementia (Chidai 痴呆)

- Treatment

    1) Above the eyebrow （ Between DU-24
    (Shenting 神庭） and EX-HN3 (Yintang 印堂)
    2) DU-20 (Baihui 百会) - DU21 (Qianding 前顶)
    zone
    3) BL-3 (Meichong 眉冲)

4) DU-19 (Houding 后顶) - DU-18 (Qiangjiang 强间) zone

5) DU-15 (Yamen 哑门)-BL-10 (Tianzhu 天柱)-SJ-17 (Yifeng 翳风) zone

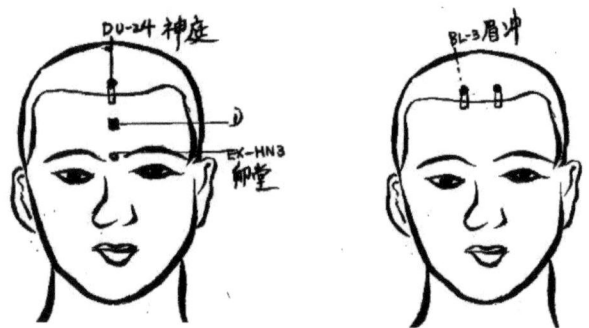

2-9 Headache (Toutong 头痛)

- Treatment

  Headache in the parietal region, upper two-fifths of the sensory area on both sides.

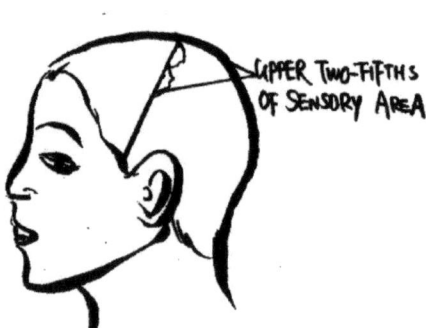

III. Disturbance of urination

3-1 Cortical frequent urination (Picent niaopin Picent 皮层尿频)

- Symptom
  Inflexibility of foot and urination.

- Treatment
  Motor and sensory area of foot on both sides.

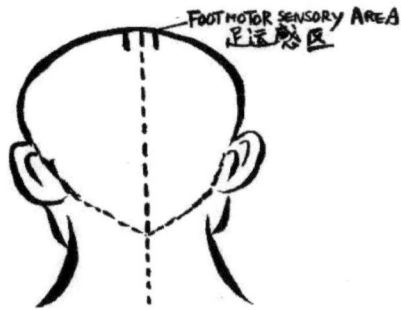

3-2 Cortical incontinence of urine (Pizhixingniaoshijin 皮质性尿失禁)

- Symptom
  Remain urination without notice.

- Treatment

Motor and sensory area of foot on both sides.

3-3 Mellitus insipidus (Niaobengzheng 尿崩症)

- Symptom
  Excessive intake water and polyuria.

- Treatment
  1) Motor and sensory area of foot.
  2) Reproductive area on both sides.

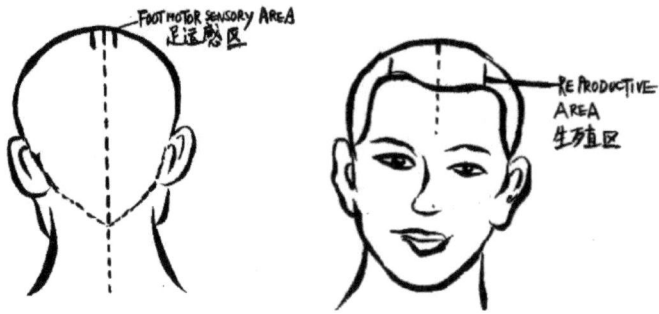

IV. Genecology
4-1 Irregular menstruation (Yuejingbutiao 月经不调)

- Symptom
  1) Precede menstrual flow.
  2) Delayed menstrual flow.

3) Disorder of menstrual flow.

- Treatment
  1) DU-20 (Baihui 百会) – DU21 (Qianding 前顶) zone.
  2) ST-8 (Touwei 头维)

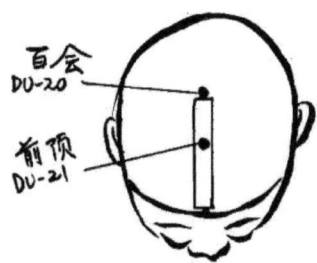 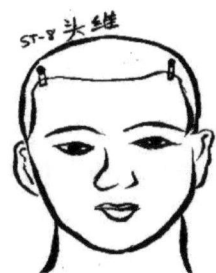

4-2 Dysmenorrhoea (Tongjing 痛经)

- Symptom
  1) Status of Qi and Blood
  2) Liver and Kidney Yin deficiency

- Behandling
  1) DU-20 (Baihui 百会) – DU-21 (Qianding 前顶) zone
  2) ST-8 (Towei 头维)

4-3 Amenorrhoea (Bijing 闭经)

- Symptom
  1) Blood stasis
  2) Blood deficiency

- Treatment
  1) DU-20 (Baihui 百会) – DU-21 (Qianding 前顶) zone
  2) ST-8 (Towei 头维)

4-4 Menopause (Juejing 绝经)

It is usually seen in woman who is about 55 years old, and at the period before or of menstruation.

- Manifestation
  The manifestations are sudden termination or disorder of menstruation, and flushed face, lassitude, sweating, listlessness, depression, irritability, insomnia, palpitation.

- Treatment
  1) DU-24 (Shenting 神庭)
  2) BL-3 (Meichong 眉冲)
  3) DU-20 (Baihui 百会) – DU21 (Qianding 前顶) zone

4) DU-15 (Yamen 哑门) -SJ-17 (Yifeng 翳风) - BL-10 (Tianzhu 天柱) zone

V. Hypertension (Gaoxieya 高血压)

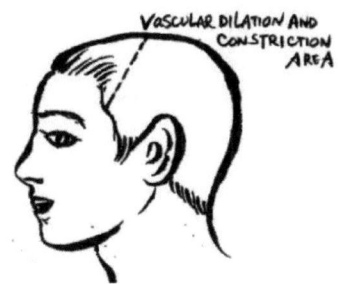

- Treatment
  Upper half of the vascular dilation and constriction area on both sides.

VI. Respiratory system diseases
6-1 Cold (Ganmao 感冒)

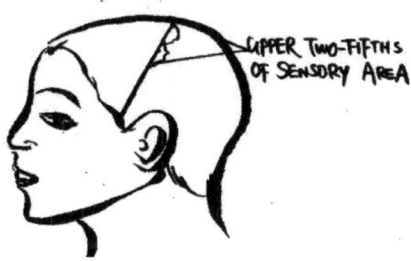

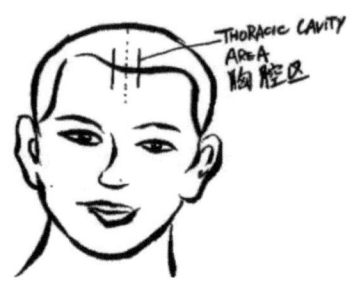

- Treatment
  1) Thoracic cavity area.
  2) Upper two-fifths of sensory area on both sides.
  3) DU-24 (Shenting 神庭)
  4) DU-20(Baihui 百会) – DU-17(Naofu 脑户) zone of 1/3.
  5) DU-15 (Yamen 哑门) -SJ-17 (Yifeng 翳风) - BL-10 (Tianzhu 天柱) 1/3 of middle zone

6-2 Bronchial Asthma (Zhiqiguanxiaochuan 支气管哮喘)

- Symptom
  Shortness of breath, wheezing, chest distress, cough with sputum, edema secretion of mucosa.
- Treatment

1) Thoracic cavity area on both sides. (BL-3 Meichong 眉冲)

2) Du-24 (Shenting 神庭)

3) DU-20 (Baihui 百会) - DU21 (Qianding 前顶) zone

4) DU-20 (Baihui 百会) - DU-19 (Houding 后顶) zone

5) DU-19 (Houding 后顶) - DU-18 (Qiangjian 强间) zone

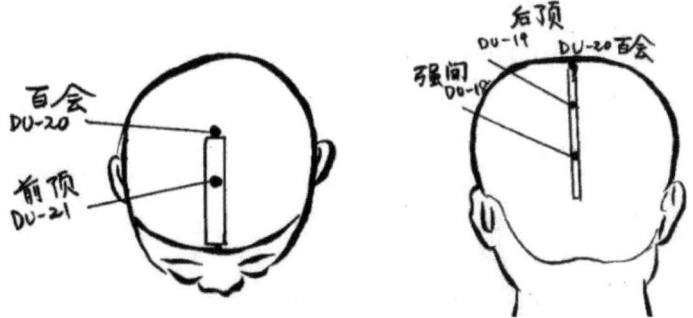

6-3 Bronchitis (Zhiqiguanyan 支气管炎)

- Treatment

    1) Thoracic cavity area on both sides. BL-3 (Meichong 眉冲)

    2) DU-24 (Shenting 神庭)

3) GB-15 (Toulinqi 头临泣)

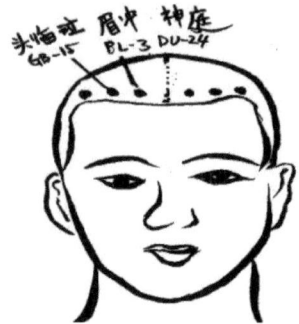

VII. Male Sexual Disorders
7-1 Emission (Paifang 排放)

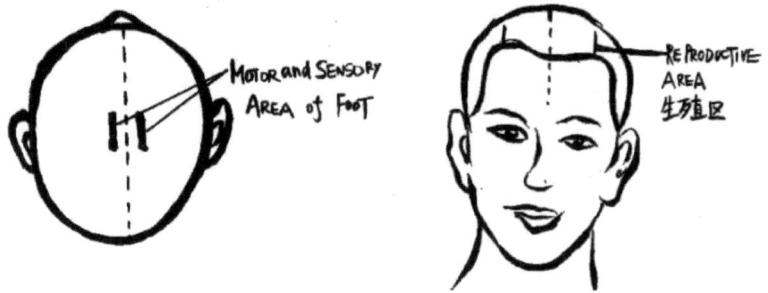

- Treatment
  1) Motor and sensory area of foot.
  2) Reproductive area on both sides.

7-2 Impotence (Yangwei 阳痿)

- Treatment
  1) Motor and sensory area of foot.
  2) Reproductive area on both sides.

VIII. Diarrhoea

8-1 Abdominal pain and diarrhoea (Futong he fuxie 腹痛和腹泻)

- Treatment
  1) Motor and sensory area of foot.
  2) Reproductive area on both sides.

8-2 Constipation (Bianmi 便秘)

- Treatment
  1) DU-20 (Baihui 百会) – DU-21 (Tianding 前顶) zone
  2) GB-15 (Toulinqi 头临泣)

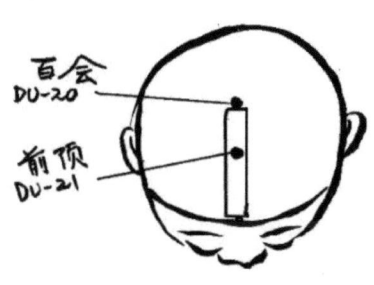 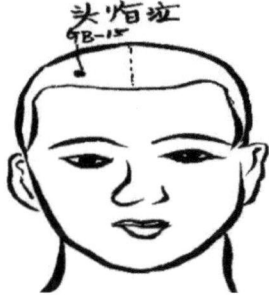

IX. Diabetes Mellitus (Tangniaobing 糖尿病)

9-1 Diabetes Mellitus

- Symptom
  Polyuria, increased water and food intake, fatigue and emaciation.

- Treatment
  1) Motor and sensory area of foot.
  2) Reproductive area on both sides.

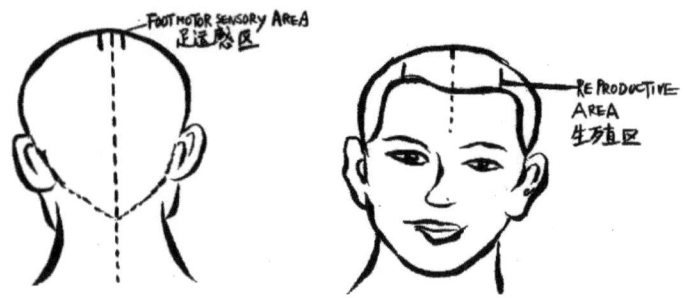

9-2 Obesity (Feipang 肥胖)

- Symptom
  Patients have visible fat accumulations in the neck, lower abdomen and buttock. Mild obese patients do not have signs of symptom, but severe patients have metabolic disturbances of

aversion to heat, profuse sweating, fatigue, dizziness, headache, palpitation.

- Treatment
  1) DU-20 (Baihui 百会) – DU-21 (Tianding 前顶) zone
  2) GB-15 (Toulinqi 头临泣)
  3) ST-8 (Touwei 头维)

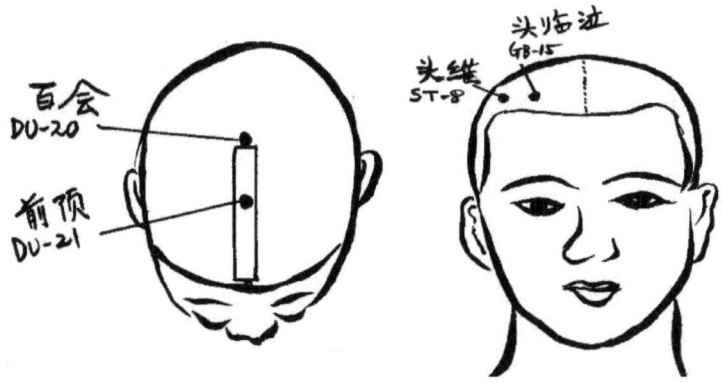

X. Bone diseases
10-1 Cervical spondylopathy (Jingchuibing 颈椎病)

- Symptom
  Pain in the head, neck, arm, hand and chest and difficult to move of the limbs.

- Treatment
  1) Motor and sensory area of foot.
  2) Upper two-fifths of the sensory area on the opposite side of the symptoms. Both sides for with symptoms on both sides.
  3) DU-20(Baihui 百会) – DU-17(Naofu 脑户) zone of 1/3.
  4) DU-15 (Yamen 哑门) -SJ-17 (Yifeng 翳风) - BL-10 (Tianzhu 天柱) 1/3 of middle zone.

10-2 Numbness in both arms (Mamu 麻木)

- Treatment
  Motor and sensory area of foot on both sides.

10-3 Lumbar spinal canal stenosis (Yaochuiguanxiazhaizheng 腰椎管狭窄症)

- Treatment
  1) Motor and sensory area of foot.
  2) Upper two-fifths of the sensory area on the opposite side of the symptoms. On both sides for symptoms on both sides.

10-4 Lumbago and pain in the legs (Yaotong he tuitong 腰痛和腿痛)

- Treatment
  1) Motor and sensory area of foot.
  2) Upper two-fifths of the sensory area on both sides.

10-5 Pain in Lumbar and sacral region (Yaobu he dibuteng 腰部和骶部疼痛)

- Treatment
  1) Motor and sensory area of foot.
  2) upper two-fifths of the sensory area on both sides.

XI. Dermatological Diseases

11-1 Cutaneous pruritus (Pifusaoyang 皮肤瘙痒)

- Symptom
  Itching of body.

- Treatment

1) Motor and sensory area of foot.

2) Upper two-fifths of the sensory area on both sides.

11-2 Contact dermatitis (Jiechuxingpiyan 接触性皮炎)

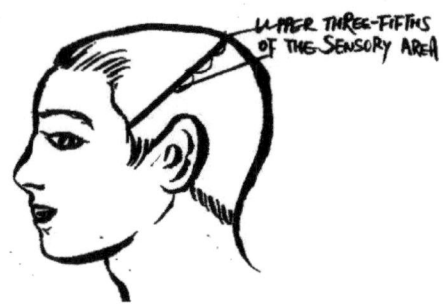

- Symptom
  Acute inflammation caused by contact with some irritative matters, and includes by animals, plants, chemicals.

- Treatment
  1) Motor and sensory area of foot.
  2) Upper three-fifths of the sensory area on the opposite side of the lesions. On both sides if the lesions are on both sides of the body.

11-3 Neurodermatitis (Shenjingxingpiyan 神经性皮炎)

- Symptom
  Chronic dermatitis which is by local itching and thickened skin and polygonal papules.

- Treatment
  1) Motor and sensory area of foot.
  2) Upper three-fifths of the sensory area on the opposite side of the lesions. If the lesions are on both sides, select the above area on both sides.

11-4 Itching and roughness of skin over both wrists (Liangshouwanpifufayangcucao 两手腕皮肤发痒粗糙)

- Treatment
  1) Motor and sensory area of foot.
  2) Upper two-fifths of sensory area on both sides.

11-5 Alopecia areata (Bantu 斑秃)

- Symptom
  Suddenly local loss of hair.

- Treatment
  1) Motor and sensory area of foot.
  2) Upper three-fifths of sensory area on both sides.

11-6 Madarosis (Jiemaotuoluo 睫毛脱落)

- Symptom
  Loss of eyebrows and eyelashes.

- Treatment
  1) Motor and sensory area of foot.
  2) Sensory area on both sides.

11-7 Urticaria (Xunmazhen 荨麻疹)

It is abrupt onset with itching flat-topped wheals of various size on the skin. In TCM, it calls Wind Wheal.

- Manifestation
  1. Wind Heat

The manifestations are red rashes, severe itching, rapid pulse.

2. Wind Damp
The manifestations are Light red or white rashes superficial and rapid pulse.
3. Accumulation of Heat in the Stomach and Intestine
The manifestations are, red rashes, abdominal pain, constipation, diarrhea, thin yellow tongue coating, and rapid pulse.

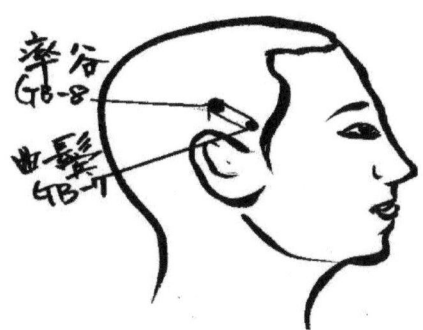

- Treatment
  1) DU-20 (Baihui 百会) - DU21 (Qianding 前顶) zone.
  2) BL-3 (Meichong 眉冲).
  3) GB-8 (Shuaigu 率谷) – GB-7 (Qubin 曲鬓) above 1/5 and middle of 2/5 zone.

11-8 Acne (Cuochuang 痤疮)

- Manifestation

  Acne is most cases on face, which may release white bodies upon squeezing. This follows by the formation of small pustules with tidal feverish, itching and pain sensation.

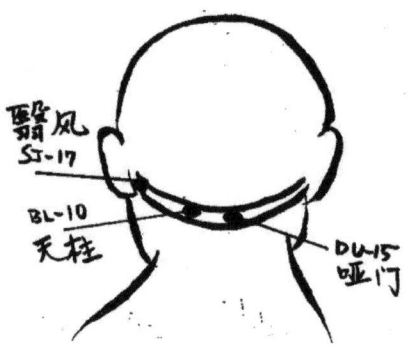

- Treatment

  1) DU-24 (Shenting 神庭)

  2) GB-15 (Toulinqi 头临泣)

  3) ST-8 (Touwei 头维)

  4) DU-15 (Yamen 哑门)-BL-10 (Tianzhu 天柱)-SJ-17 (Yifeng 翳风) 1/3 zone

XII. Diseases of Ears and Eyes

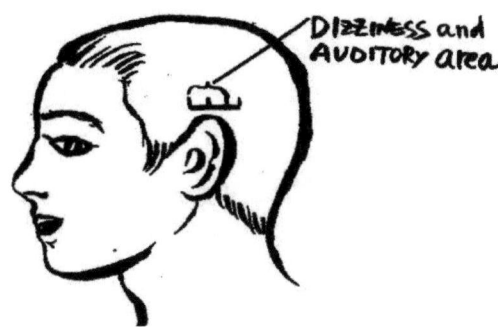

12-1 Vertigo (Xuanyun 眩晕)

- Symptom
  1. Hyperactivity of Liver Yang
  The manifestations are tinnitus, nausea, backache disturbed sleep, flushed face, congested eyes, red tongue proper with thin yellow coating, wiry rapid pulse.

  2. Qi and Blood Deficiency
  The manifestations are palpitation, insomnia, pale complexion, pale complexion, poor appetite, pale tongue proper, weak pulse.

  3. Phlegm-Damp obstruction in the interior
  The manifestations are lassitude, fullness in the chest and epigastrium, heaviness of head,

vomiting, white and sticky tongue, rolling pulse.

- Treatment
Dizziness and auditory area on both sides.

12-2 Dizziness (Touyun 头晕)

- Symptom
feeling faint, woozy, weak or unsteady.
- Treatment
Dizziness and auditory area on both sides.

12-3 Deafness (Erlong 耳聋)

Deafness refers to loss of hearing and low degree of hearing. It is gradually intensified deafness.

- Symptom
1. Excess of Liver and Gallbladder.
   The manifestations are irritability, heavy sensation of the head, bitter taste in mouth, red tongue with yellow coating rapid wiry pulse.

2. Deficiency of Kidney Essence
   It is gradually intensified deafness.

The manifestations are dizziness, lassitude, low back pain, insomnia, red tongue with little coating, and weak thready pulse.
- Treatment
Dizziness and auditory area on both sides.

12-4 Tinnitus (Erming 耳鸣)

Tinnitus is characterized by continuous ringing of the ear.
- Symptom
1. Excess of Liver and Gallbladder.
   It is continuous ringing in the ear and there is no relieving.
2. Deficiency of Kidney Essence
   It is intermittent ringing and it becomes aggravated after stress and strain, but it is alleviated by pressure.

- Treatment
Dizziness and auditory area on both sides.

12-5 Rhinitis (Biyan 鼻炎)

This is by nasal obstruction and nasal secretion.

- Symptom

This is induced by the exogenous Wind-Cold or Wind-Heat, improper diet, and the manifestations are nasal secretion of thick and yellow mucosa.

- Treatment
  1) DU-24 (Shenting 神庭)
  2) BL-3 (Meichong 眉冲)
  3) Above the eyeblow (Between DU-24 (Shenting 神庭) and EX-HN3 (Yintang 印堂)

12-6 Tonsilitis (Biantaotiyan 扁桃体炎)

It is caused by inflammation by the invasion of streptococcus and staphylococcus.

- Symptom
  The symptom is marked by swelling, pain, fever, headache.
  1. Wind-Heat
  2. Deficiency of Kidney Yin

- Treatment
  1) DU-24 (Shenting 神庭)
  2) BL-3 (Meichong 眉冲)

12-7 Myopia (Jinshi 近视)

It is characterized in that the eyes can see near objects but not distant.

- Manifestation
  It is clear for near objects but blurred vision for distant which may be accompanied by tinnitus, insomnia, dizziness, pale tongue, and weak thready pulse.

- Treatment
  1) DU-24 (Shenting 神庭)
  2) DU-24 (Shenting 神庭) – (DU-2 前顶) 1/3 zone
  3) DU-20 (Baihui 百会) – DU-17 (Naohu 脑户) above of 1/3 and down of 1/3 zone
  4) DU-15 (Yamen 哑门) - BL-10 (Tianzhu 天柱) - SJ-17 (Yifeng 翳风) zone

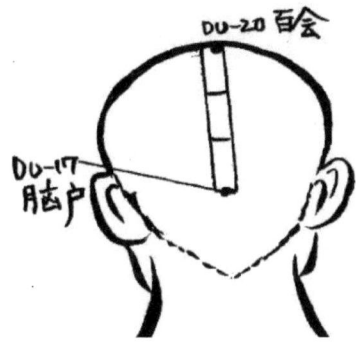

12-8 Cataract (Baineizhang 白内障)

This is divided to Congenital and Acquired.

- Symptom
(1) Congenital
(2) Acquired
  This is mainly affecting those over 50 years old and is characterized by chronic disorder in both eyes. It causes deficiency Liver, Kidney, Spleen, Stomach, Yin deficiency and is failure the essence and blood to prevent eye malnourishment.

- Treatment
  1) DU-20 (Baihui 百会) – DU-17 (Naohu 脑户) down of 1/3
  2) DU-24 (Shenting 神庭)

12-9 Conjunctivis (Jiemoyan 结膜炎)

Congestion, swelling and pain of the eye in acute.

- Symptom
  Invasion for exogenous wind-heat.
  The manifestations are swelling and pain, burning sensation in the eyelids, and this is

caused by excessive fire in the Liver and
Gallbladder, bitter taste in the mouth,
dizziness, red tongue with yellow coating, and
rapid wiry pulse.

- Treatment
  1) DU-20 (Baihui 百会) – DU-17 (Naohu 脑户)
  above of 1/3 and down of 1/3.
  2) DU-24 (Shenting 神庭).

References 参考文献

1. Jie Yan, Skills with Illustrations of Chinese Acupuncture and Moxibution, 1991.

2. Chaoyang Wang, Touzhen Yundong Liaofa, 2006.

3. Jiao Shunfa, Scalp Acupuncture and Clinical Cases, 1990.

4. Wang Lingli, Chinese Acupuncture and Moxibution, 2002.

5. Medical Dictionary, Brodmann